THIS BOOK BELONGS TO

Date: ____________________

Time	Food	Category	Notes
Water	☐ ☐ ☐ ☐ ☐ ☐ ☐ ☐ ☐ ☐ ☐		

Date: ______________________

Time	Food	Category	Notes
Water	☐ ☐ ☐ ☐ ☐ ☐ ☐ ☐ ☐ ☐ ☐		

Date: ____________________

Time	Food	Category	Notes
Water	☐ ☐ ☐ ☐ ☐ ☐ ☐ ☐ ☐ ☐ ☐		

Date: ______________________________

Time	Food	Category	Notes

Water ☐ ☐ ☐ ☐ ☐ ☐ ☐ ☐ ☐ ☐ ☐

Date: ____________________

Time	Food	Category	Notes
Water	☐ ☐ ☐ ☐ ☐ ☐ ☐ ☐ ☐ ☐ ☐		

Date: ______________________

Time	Food	Category	Notes
Water	☐ ☐ ☐ ☐ ☐ ☐ ☐ ☐ ☐ ☐ ☐		

Date: ____________________

Time	Food	Category	Notes
Water	☐ ☐ ☐ ☐ ☐ ☐ ☐ ☐ ☐ ☐ ☐		

Date: ____________________________

Time	Food	Category	Notes
Water	☐ ☐ ☐ ☐ ☐ ☐ ☐ ☐ ☐ ☐ ☐		

Date: ______________________

Time	Food	Category	Notes

Water ☐ ☐ ☐ ☐ ☐ ☐ ☐ ☐ ☐ ☐ ☐

Date: ____________________

Time	Food	Category	Notes
Water	☐ ☐ ☐ ☐ ☐ ☐ ☐ ☐ ☐ ☐ ☐		

Date: ____________________

Time	Food	Category	Notes
Water	☐ ☐ ☐ ☐ ☐ ☐ ☐ ☐ ☐ ☐ ☐		

Date: ____________________

Time	Food	Category	Notes
Water	☐ ☐ ☐ ☐ ☐ ☐ ☐ ☐ ☐ ☐ ☐		

Date: ____________________

Time	Food	Category	Notes
Water	☐ ☐ ☐ ☐ ☐ ☐ ☐ ☐ ☐ ☐ ☐		

Date: ______________________

Time	Food	Category	Notes

Water	☐	☐	☐	☐	☐	☐	☐	☐	☐	☐	☐

Date: ______________________

Time	Food	Category	Notes
Water	☐ ☐ ☐ ☐ ☐ ☐ ☐ ☐ ☐ ☐ ☐		

Date: ____________________

Time	Food	Category	Notes
Water	☐ ☐ ☐ ☐ ☐ ☐ ☐ ☐ ☐ ☐ ☐		

Date: ____________________

Time	Food	Category	Notes
Water	☐ ☐ ☐ ☐ ☐ ☐ ☐ ☐ ☐ ☐ ☐		

Date: ______________________

Time	Food	Category	Notes
Water	☐ ☐ ☐ ☐ ☐ ☐ ☐ ☐ ☐ ☐ ☐		

Date: ____________________

Time	Food	Category	Notes
Water	☐ ☐ ☐ ☐ ☐ ☐ ☐ ☐ ☐ ☐ ☐		

Date: ____________________

Time	Food	Category	Notes
Water	☐ ☐ ☐ ☐ ☐ ☐ ☐ ☐ ☐ ☐ ☐		

Date: ______________________

Time	Food	Category	Notes
Water	☐ ☐ ☐ ☐ ☐ ☐ ☐ ☐ ☐ ☐ ☐		

Date: ____________________

Time	Food	Category	Notes
Water	☐ ☐ ☐ ☐ ☐ ☐ ☐ ☐ ☐ ☐ ☐		

Date: ____________________

Time	Food	Category	Notes
Water	☐ ☐ ☐ ☐ ☐ ☐ ☐ ☐ ☐ ☐ ☐		

Date: ______________________________

Time	Food	Category	Notes
Water	☐ ☐ ☐ ☐ ☐ ☐ ☐ ☐ ☐ ☐ ☐		

Date: ____________________

Time	Food	Category	Notes
Water	☐ ☐ ☐ ☐ ☐ ☐ ☐ ☐ ☐ ☐ ☐		

Date: ______________________________

Time	Food	Category	Notes
Water	☐ ☐ ☐ ☐ ☐ ☐ ☐ ☐ ☐ ☐ ☐		

Date: ___________________________

Time	Food	Category	Notes
Water	☐ ☐ ☐ ☐ ☐ ☐ ☐ ☐ ☐ ☐ ☐		

Date: ______________________

Time	Food	Category	Notes
Water	☐ ☐ ☐ ☐ ☐ ☐ ☐ ☐ ☐ ☐ ☐		

Date: ____________________

Time	Food	Category	Notes
Water	☐ ☐ ☐ ☐ ☐ ☐ ☐ ☐ ☐ ☐ ☐		

Date: ______________________

Time	Food	Category	Notes
Water	☐ ☐ ☐ ☐ ☐ ☐ ☐ ☐ ☐ ☐ ☐		

Date: ______________________

Time	Food	Category	Notes
Water	☐ ☐ ☐ ☐ ☐ ☐ ☐ ☐ ☐ ☐ ☐		

Date: ______________________

Time	Food	Category	Notes
Water	☐ ☐ ☐ ☐ ☐ ☐ ☐ ☐ ☐ ☐ ☐		

Date: ____________________

Time	Food	Category	Notes
Water	☐ ☐ ☐ ☐ ☐ ☐ ☐ ☐ ☐ ☐ ☐		

Date: ______________________

Time	Food	Category	Notes
Water	☐ ☐ ☐ ☐ ☐ ☐ ☐ ☐ ☐ ☐ ☐		

Date: ____________________

Time	Food	Category	Notes
Water	☐ ☐ ☐ ☐ ☐ ☐ ☐ ☐ ☐ ☐ ☐		

Date: ______________________________

Time	Food	Category	Notes
Water	☐ ☐ ☐ ☐ ☐ ☐ ☐ ☐ ☐ ☐ ☐		

Date: ____________________

Time	Food	Category	Notes
Water	☐ ☐ ☐ ☐ ☐ ☐ ☐ ☐ ☐ ☐ ☐		

Date: ____________________________

Time	Food	Category	Notes

Water	☐ ☐ ☐ ☐ ☐ ☐ ☐ ☐ ☐ ☐ ☐

Date: ______________________

Time	Food	Category	Notes
Water	☐ ☐ ☐ ☐ ☐ ☐ ☐ ☐ ☐ ☐ ☐		

Date: ____________________

Time	Food	Category	Notes
Water	☐ ☐ ☐ ☐ ☐ ☐ ☐ ☐ ☐ ☐ ☐		

Date: ______________________

Time	Food	Category	Notes
Water	☐ ☐ ☐ ☐ ☐ ☐ ☐ ☐ ☐ ☐ ☐		

Date: ______________________

Time	Food	Category	Notes
Water	☐ ☐ ☐ ☐ ☐ ☐ ☐ ☐ ☐ ☐ ☐		

Date: ____________________________

Time	Food	Category	Notes

Water ☐ ☐ ☐ ☐ ☐ ☐ ☐ ☐ ☐ ☐ ☐

Date: ______________________

Time	Food	Category	Notes
Water	☐ ☐ ☐ ☐ ☐ ☐ ☐ ☐ ☐ ☐ ☐		

Date: ____________________

Time	Food	Category	Notes
Water	☐ ☐ ☐ ☐ ☐ ☐ ☐ ☐ ☐ ☐ ☐		

Date: ______________________________

Time	Food	Category	Notes
Water	☐ ☐ ☐ ☐ ☐ ☐ ☐ ☐ ☐ ☐ ☐		

Date: ______________________

Time	Food	Category	Notes

Water	☐	☐	☐	☐	☐	☐	☐	☐	☐	☐	☐

Date: ____________________

Time	Food	Category	Notes
Water	☐ ☐ ☐ ☐ ☐ ☐ ☐ ☐ ☐ ☐ ☐		

Date: ____________________

Time	Food	Category	Notes
Water	☐ ☐ ☐ ☐ ☐ ☐ ☐ ☐ ☐ ☐ ☐		

Date: ____________________________

Time	Food	Category	Notes
Water	☐ ☐ ☐ ☐ ☐ ☐ ☐ ☐ ☐ ☐ ☐		

Date: ______________________

Time	Food	Category	Notes
Water	☐ ☐ ☐ ☐ ☐ ☐ ☐ ☐ ☐ ☐ ☐		

Date: ______________________

Time	Food	Category	Notes
Water	☐ ☐ ☐ ☐ ☐ ☐ ☐ ☐ ☐ ☐ ☐		

Date: ____________________

Time	Food	Category	Notes
Water	☐ ☐ ☐ ☐ ☐ ☐ ☐ ☐ ☐ ☐ ☐		

Date: ____________________

Time	Food	Category	Notes
Water	☐ ☐ ☐ ☐ ☐ ☐ ☐ ☐ ☐ ☐ ☐		

Date: ____________________

Time	Food	Category	Notes
Water	☐ ☐ ☐ ☐ ☐ ☐ ☐ ☐ ☐ ☐ ☐		

Date: ______________________

Time	Food	Category	Notes
Water	☐ ☐ ☐ ☐ ☐ ☐ ☐ ☐ ☐ ☐ ☐		

Date: ______________________

Time	Food	Category	Notes
Water	☐ ☐ ☐ ☐ ☐ ☐ ☐ ☐ ☐ ☐ ☐		

Date: ____________________________

Time	Food	Category	Notes
Water	☐ ☐ ☐ ☐ ☐ ☐ ☐ ☐ ☐ ☐ ☐		

Date: ____________________

Time	Food	Category	Notes
Water	☐ ☐ ☐ ☐ ☐ ☐ ☐ ☐ ☐ ☐ ☐		

Date: ____________________________

Time	Food	Category	Notes
Water	☐ ☐ ☐ ☐ ☐ ☐ ☐ ☐ ☐ ☐ ☐		

Date: ____________________

Time	Food	Category	Notes
Water	☐ ☐ ☐ ☐ ☐ ☐ ☐ ☐ ☐ ☐ ☐		

Date: ______________________

Time	Food	Category	Notes
Water	☐ ☐ ☐ ☐ ☐ ☐ ☐ ☐ ☐ ☐ ☐		

Date: ______________________

Time	Food	Category	Notes
Water	☐ ☐ ☐ ☐ ☐ ☐ ☐ ☐ ☐ ☐ ☐		

Date: ______________________

Time	Food	Category	Notes
Water	☐ ☐ ☐ ☐ ☐ ☐ ☐ ☐ ☐ ☐ ☐		

Date: ____________________

Time	Food	Category	Notes
Water	☐ ☐ ☐ ☐ ☐ ☐ ☐ ☐ ☐ ☐ ☐		

Date: ____________________

Time	Food	Category	Notes
Water	☐ ☐ ☐ ☐ ☐ ☐ ☐ ☐ ☐ ☐ ☐		

Date: ______________________

Time	Food	Category	Notes
Water	☐ ☐ ☐ ☐ ☐ ☐ ☐ ☐ ☐ ☐ ☐		

Date: ____________________

Time	Food	Category	Notes
Water	☐ ☐ ☐ ☐ ☐ ☐ ☐ ☐ ☐ ☐ ☐		

Date: ______________________

Time	Food	Category	Notes
Water	☐ ☐ ☐ ☐ ☐ ☐ ☐ ☐ ☐ ☐ ☐		

Date: ____________________________

Time	Food	Category	Notes
Water	☐ ☐ ☐ ☐ ☐ ☐ ☐ ☐ ☐ ☐ ☐		

Date: ______________________________

Time	Food	Category	Notes
Water	☐ ☐ ☐ ☐ ☐ ☐ ☐ ☐ ☐ ☐ ☐		

Date: ______________________

Time	Food	Category	Notes
Water	☐ ☐ ☐ ☐ ☐ ☐ ☐ ☐ ☐ ☐ ☐		

Date: ______________________

Time	Food	Category	Notes
Water	☐ ☐ ☐ ☐ ☐ ☐ ☐ ☐ ☐ ☐ ☐		

Date: ______________________________

Time	Food	Category	Notes
Water	☐ ☐ ☐ ☐ ☐ ☐ ☐ ☐ ☐ ☐ ☐		

Date: ______________________

Time	Food	Category	Notes
Water	☐ ☐ ☐ ☐ ☐ ☐ ☐ ☐ ☐ ☐ ☐		

Date: ______________________

Time	Food	Category	Notes
Water	☐ ☐ ☐ ☐ ☐ ☐ ☐ ☐ ☐ ☐ ☐		

Date: ____________________

Time	Food	Category	Notes
Water	☐ ☐ ☐ ☐ ☐ ☐ ☐ ☐ ☐ ☐ ☐		

Date: ____________________

Time	Food	Category	Notes
Water	☐ ☐ ☐ ☐ ☐ ☐ ☐ ☐ ☐ ☐ ☐		

Date: ___________________________

Time	Food	Category	Notes
Water	☐ ☐ ☐ ☐ ☐ ☐ ☐ ☐ ☐ ☐ ☐		

Date: ____________________

Time	Food	Category	Notes
Water	☐ ☐ ☐ ☐ ☐ ☐ ☐ ☐ ☐ ☐ ☐		

Date: ______________________

Time	Food	Category	Notes
Water	☐ ☐ ☐ ☐ ☐ ☐ ☐ ☐ ☐ ☐ ☐		

Date: ______________________

Time	Food	Category	Notes
Water	☐ ☐ ☐ ☐ ☐ ☐ ☐ ☐ ☐ ☐ ☐		

Date: ____________________

Time	Food	Category	Notes
Water	☐ ☐ ☐ ☐ ☐ ☐ ☐ ☐ ☐ ☐ ☐		

Date: ______________________

Time	Food	Category	Notes
Water	☐ ☐ ☐ ☐ ☐ ☐ ☐ ☐ ☐ ☐ ☐		

Date: ______________________

Time	Food	Category	Notes
Water	☐ ☐ ☐ ☐ ☐ ☐ ☐ ☐ ☐ ☐ ☐		

Date: ____________________

Time	Food	Category	Notes
Water	☐ ☐ ☐ ☐ ☐ ☐ ☐ ☐ ☐ ☐ ☐		

Date: ____________________

Time	Food	Category	Notes
Water	☐ ☐ ☐ ☐ ☐ ☐ ☐ ☐ ☐ ☐ ☐		

Date: ____________________

Time	Food	Category	Notes

Water ☐ ☐ ☐ ☐ ☐ ☐ ☐ ☐ ☐ ☐ ☐

Date: ____________________

Time	Food	Category	Notes
Water	☐ ☐ ☐ ☐ ☐ ☐ ☐ ☐ ☐ ☐ ☐		

Date: ______________________

Time	Food	Category	Notes
Water	☐ ☐ ☐ ☐ ☐ ☐ ☐ ☐ ☐ ☐ ☐		

Date: ______________________

Time	Food	Category	Notes
Water	☐ ☐ ☐ ☐ ☐ ☐ ☐ ☐ ☐ ☐ ☐		

Date: ______________________

Time	Food	Category	Notes
Water	☐ ☐ ☐ ☐ ☐ ☐ ☐ ☐ ☐ ☐ ☐		

Date: ______________________

Time	Food	Category	Notes
Water	☐ ☐ ☐ ☐ ☐ ☐ ☐ ☐ ☐ ☐ ☐		

Date: ______________________

Time	Food	Category	Notes
Water	☐ ☐ ☐ ☐ ☐ ☐ ☐ ☐ ☐ ☐ ☐		

Date: ____________________

Time	Food	Category	Notes
Water	☐ ☐ ☐ ☐ ☐ ☐ ☐ ☐ ☐ ☐ ☐		

Date: ______________________

Time	Food	Category	Notes
Water	☐ ☐ ☐ ☐ ☐ ☐ ☐ ☐ ☐ ☐ ☐		

Date: ____________________

Time	Food	Category	Notes
Water	☐ ☐ ☐ ☐ ☐ ☐ ☐ ☐ ☐ ☐ ☐		

Date: ______________________

Time	Food	Category	Notes
Water	☐ ☐ ☐ ☐ ☐ ☐ ☐ ☐ ☐ ☐ ☐		

Date: ____________________

Time	Food	Category	Notes
Water	☐ ☐ ☐ ☐ ☐ ☐ ☐ ☐ ☐ ☐ ☐		

Date: ____________________

Time	Food	Category	Notes
Water	☐ ☐ ☐ ☐ ☐ ☐ ☐ ☐ ☐ ☐ ☐		

Date: ______________________

Time	Food	Category	Notes
Water	☐ ☐ ☐ ☐ ☐ ☐ ☐ ☐ ☐ ☐ ☐		

Date: ____________________

Time	Food	Category	Notes
Water	☐ ☐ ☐ ☐ ☐ ☐ ☐ ☐ ☐ ☐ ☐		

Date: ____________________

Time	Food	Category	Notes
Water	☐ ☐ ☐ ☐ ☐ ☐ ☐ ☐ ☐ ☐ ☐		

Date: ______________________

Time	Food	Category	Notes
Water	☐ ☐ ☐ ☐ ☐ ☐ ☐ ☐ ☐ ☐ ☐		

Date: ____________________

Time	Food	Category	Notes
Water	☐ ☐ ☐ ☐ ☐ ☐ ☐ ☐ ☐ ☐ ☐		

Date: ______________________

Time	Food	Category	Notes
Water	☐ ☐ ☐ ☐ ☐ ☐ ☐ ☐ ☐ ☐ ☐		

Date: ______________________

Time	Food	Category	Notes
Water	☐ ☐ ☐ ☐ ☐ ☐ ☐ ☐ ☐ ☐ ☐		

Date: ____________________

Time	Food	Category	Notes
Water	☐ ☐ ☐ ☐ ☐ ☐ ☐ ☐ ☐ ☐ ☐		

Date: ____________________

Time	Food	Category	Notes
Water	☐ ☐ ☐ ☐ ☐ ☐ ☐ ☐ ☐ ☐ ☐		

www.ingramcontent.com/pod-product-compliance
Lightning Source LLC
Chambersburg PA
CBHW060417290526
45791CB00002B/784
* 9 7 8 1 0 7 6 9 2 0 8 9 8 *